THE NEW MENOPAUSE DIET COOKBOOK

Nourishing Recipes to Support Your Changing Body

Juliet Michael James

DISCLAIMER

The recipes provided in this cookbook are intended for informational purposes only. While every effort has been made to ensure accuracy, the author and publisher do not assume any responsibility for any individual's personal health, dietary restrictions, allergies, or cooking abilities. The author and publisher disclaim any liability for any loss or damage resulting from the use of the recipes contained within this cookbook. Cooking involves inherent risks, and readers should exercise caution, especially when dealing with heat, sharp utensils, and handling of ingredients. By using this cookbook, you agree that the author and publisher are not responsible or liable for any personal injury, property damage, or other damages that may result from the use of the information, recipes, or techniques presented herein.

TABLE OF CONTENTS

Chapter 1

Introduction to Menopause and Nutrition

AS A WOMAN, YOU'RE NO STRANGER TO THE VARIOUS PHASES of life that come with unique challenges and transitions. One such pivotal stage is menopause – a natural biological process that marks the end of your reproductive years. While this transition is often associated with a range of physical and emotional symptoms, it's important to understand that menopause is a natural part of aging, not a disorder or a disease.

Menopause typically occurs between the ages of 45 and 55, although some women may experience it earlier or later. During this time, your ovaries gradually produce less estrogen and progesterone, the two main hormones responsible for regulating your menstrual cycle. As these hormone levels fluctuate and eventually decline, you may experience a variety of symptoms that can impact your daily life.

Common Menopause Symptoms

1. Hot flashes: These sudden feelings of intense heat, often accompanied by sweating and a rapid heartbeat, are one of the most well-known menopausal symptoms. Hot flashes can occur at any time, day or night, and can range from mild to severe.

2. Night sweats: Similar to hot flashes, night sweats can disrupt your sleep patterns, leaving you feeling fatigued and irritable during the day.

3. Mood changes: The hormonal shifts during menopause can affect your mood, leading to irritability, anxiety, and even depression in some cases.

4. Weight gain: Many women report gaining weight, particularly around the abdominal area, during and after menopause. This can be attributed to a combination of hormonal changes, age-related metabolic slowdown, and lifestyle factors.

5. Vaginal dryness: Decreased estrogen levels can cause vaginal dryness, leading to discomfort during sexual activity and an increased risk of urinary tract infections.

6. **Bone loss:** Estrogen is essential for bone density maintenance, and its decrease during menopause might heighten the risk of osteoporosis, a disease that undermines bones and increases their vulnerability to fractures.

While dealing with these symptoms during menopause might be difficult, keep in mind that every woman goes through it differently. While some people may breeze through this change with no trouble, others may discover it more troublesome. No matter what your menopausal symptoms are like, it's always empowering to know how diet and nutrition play a part.

The Power of Diet in Managing Menopause Symptoms

Diet plays a crucial role in managing menopause symptoms and maintaining overall health during this transition. By making informed dietary choices, you can alleviate many of the discomforts associated with menopause and support your body's changing needs. Here's how a well-balanced, nutrient-dense diet can help:

1. Regulating hot flashes and night sweats: Certain nutrients, such as soy is of lavones, flaxseeds, and black cohosh, have been shown to help reduce the

frequency and intensity of hot flashes and night sweats.

2. Supporting bone health: Ensuring adequate intake of calcium, vitamin D, and other bone-building nutrients can help maintain bone density and reduce the risk of osteoporosis.

3. Promoting cardiovascular health: Menopause can increase the risk of heart disease, but a diet rich in fiber, healthy fats, and antioxidants can help support heart health and manage cholesterol levels.

4. Balancing mood and reducing stress: Certain foods, like those rich in omega-3 fatty acids, can help regulate mood and reduce feelings of anxiety and depression. Additionally, a balanced diet can provide the nutrients necessary for optimal brain function and stress management.

5. Maintaining a healthy weight: By focusing on nutrient-dense, whole foods and practicing portion control, you can avoid the unwanted weight gain often associated with menopause.

In the chapters ahead, we'll dive deeper into the specific dietary recommendations and nutrient needs for managing menopause symptoms effectively. You'll discover delicious and nutritious recipes that cater to your changing body's requirements, empowering you to take control of your well-being during this transitional phase.

You should always put it at the back of your that menopause is a natural part of life, and with the right dietary approach, you can navigate this journey with grace, confidence, and a renewed sense of vitality. Embrace this new chapter and let food be your ally in managing menopause symptoms and optimizing your overall health.

Benefits of a menopause-friendly diet

Here are the key benefits of following a menopause-friendly diet:

1. Alleviating Hot Flashes and Night Sweats

Hot flashes and night sweats are among the most notorious menopause symptoms, often disrupting sleep and daily activities. A menopause-friendly diet can help alleviate these discomforts by incorporating foods rich in phytoestrogens. These plant-based compounds mimic the effects of estrogen in the body, potentially reducing the frequency and intensity of hot flashes and night sweats. Soy-based products, flaxseeds, and legumes are excellent sources of phytoestrogens.

2. Supporting Bone Health

During menopause, the decline in estrogen levels can accelerate bone loss, increasing the risk of osteoporosis. A diet abundant in calcium, vitamin D, and other bone-building nutrients is crucial for maintaining strong, healthy bones. Dairy products, leafy greens, fatty fish, and fortified foods can provide these essential nutrients. Additionally, weight-bearing exercises and strength training can further promote bone density.

3. Promoting Heart Health

Menopause is often associated with an increased risk of cardiovascular disease due to fluctuating hormone levels and other age-related factors. A menopause-friendly diet rich in fiber, healthy fats (such as those found in avocados, nuts, and fatty fish), and antioxidants can help maintain healthy cholesterol levels and support overall heart health. Incorporating fruits, vegetables, whole grains, and lean proteins can also contribute to a heart-healthy lifestyle.

4. Balancing Mood and Reducing Stress

The hormonal changes during menopause can cause mood swings, anxiety, and even depression in some women. A diet rich in omega-3 fatty acids, found in fatty fishlike salmon and walnuts, can help regulate mood and reduce inflammation. Additionally, foods high in B vitamins, such as whole grains and leafy greens, support brain function and stress management.

5. Preserving a Healthy Body Weight

Weight gain, particularly around the abdominal area, is a common concern for many women going through menopause. A menopause-friendly diet focuses on nutrient-dense, whole foods that promote satiety and support a healthy metabolism. By emphasizing portion control, high-fiber foods, lean proteins, and healthy fats, you can avoid unwanted weight gain and maintain a healthy body composition.

6. Improving Overall Well-being

A well-balanced, menopause-friendly diet provides a wide range of essential vitamins, minerals, and antioxidants that support overall health and well-being. These nutrients can help boost energy levels, improve cognitive function, and promote a stronger immune system – all crucial factors for thriving during this transitional phase of life. Adopting a menopause-friendly dietary approach is a powerful step toward managing menopause symptoms and optimizing your overall health.

By nourishing your body with the right nutrients, you can navigate this transition with confidence, vitality, and a renewed sense of well-being.

Chapter 2

The Menopause Diet Principles

As you start on this road of treating menopausal symptoms via a well-balanced diet, it's crucial to grasp the concepts that will guide your food choices. By focusing on nutrient-dense meals and eliminating or avoiding specific dietary components, you may develop a firm foundation for maximum health and well-being throughout this transitional era.

Nutrient-Dense Foods for Menopause

1. Phytoestrogen-Rich Foods

Phytoestrogens are plant-based compounds that mimic the effects of estrogen in the body. Incorporating phytoestrogen-rich foods into your diet can help alleviate menopausal symptoms like hot flashes and night sweats. Here are a few top-notch sources:

- Soy products (tofu, tempeh, edamame)
- Flaxseeds and chia seeds
- Legumes (lentils, chickpeas, beans)
- Whole grains (oats, barley, quinoa)

2. Calcium-Rich Foods

Maintaining strong bones is crucial during menopause, as the decline in estrogen levels can accelerate bone loss and increase the risk of osteoporosis. Ensure you get adequate calcium from dietary sources such as:

- Dairy products (milk, yogurt, cheese)
- Leafy green vegetables (kale, spinach, collard greens)
- Fortified plant-based milks (almond, soy, or oat milk)
- Sardines and salmon (with edible bones)

3. Vitamin D-Rich Foods

Vitamin D works in tandem with calcium to promote bone health. It also plays a role in regulating immune function and mood. Foods that are rich in vitamin D include:

- Fatty fish (salmon, tuna, mackerel)
- Egg yolks
- Fortified foods (milk, cereals, juices)
- Mushrooms (especially those exposed to UV light)

4. Omega-3 Fatty Acids

Omega-3 fatty acids are essential for maintaining cardiovascular health, reducing inflammation, and supporting cognitive function. Incorporate foods like:

- Fatty fish (salmon, mackerel, sardines)
- Walnuts and flaxseeds
- Chia seeds and hemp seeds

5. Antioxidant-Rich Foods

Antioxidants can help combat oxidative stress and inflammation, which are associated with various menopausal symptoms. Load up on:

- Berries (blueberries, raspberries, strawberries)
- Leafy greens (kale, spinach, arugula)
- Tomatoes and bell peppers
- Nuts and seeds

6. High-Fiber Foods

Fiber not only supports digestive health but can also aid in weight management and regulate blood sugar levels. Incorporate plenty of:

- Whole grains (brown rice, quinoa, oats)
- Fruits and vegetables
- Legumes (lentils, beans, peas)
- Nuts and seeds

Foods to Minimize or Avoid

While focusing on nutrient-dense foods is essential, it's also crucial to be mindful of certain dietary components that can potentially exacerbate menopausal symptoms or have negative impacts on overall health.

1. Refined Carbohydrates and Added Sugars

Refined carbohydrates and added sugars can contribute to weight gain, blood sugar imbalances, and inflammation. Limit your intake of:

- White bread, pastries, and sugary cereals
- Sodas and sugary beverages
- Candy and desserts with added sugars

2. Processed Meats

Processed meats, such as deli meats, sausages, and bacon, are often high in sodium, preservatives, and unhealthy fats. These can increase the risk of chronic diseases and contribute to weight gain.

3. Alcohol

Excessive alcohol consumption can disrupt hormone levels, interfere with sleep, and increase the risk of hot flashes. Drink in moderation if you so choose.

4. Caffeine

While moderate caffeine intake may be tolerated by some, excessive consumption can exacerbate hot flashes, anxiety, and sleep disturbances. Be mindful of your caffeine sources, such as coffee, tea, and energy drinks.

5. Fried and Highly Processed Foods

Fried foods and highly processed snacks are often high in unhealthy fats, sodium, and preservatives, which can contribute to inflammation and weight gain. Opt for healthier alternatives whenever possible.

6. Trans Fats

Trans fats, found in many commercially baked goods and fried foods, can increase the risk of heart disease and other chronic conditions. Read labels carefully and avoid foods containing partially hydrogenated oils.

By emphasizing nutrient-dense foods and reducing or eliminating potentially detrimental dietary components, you'll be well on your way to designing a menopause-friendly eating plan that supports your overall health and well-being. Remember, moderation and balance are crucial, and tiny sustainable adjustments may lead to substantial gains in managing menopausal symptoms.

Importance of balance and variety

When it comes to a menopause-friendly diet, the importance of balance and variety cannot be overstated. While focusing on nutrient-dense foods and minimizing potentially harmful dietary components is crucial, it's equally important to embrace a diverse range of wholesome options. Variety not only ensures that you're getting a wide array of essential nutrients but also adds excitement and enjoyment to your eating experience.

Achieving a balanced and varied diet during menopause involves incorporating a range of food groups, flavors, and textures. By doing so, you'll not only meet your body's changing nutritional needs but also prevent dietary boredom, which can lead to unhealthy cravings and poor adherence to your dietary goals.

Variety in Fruits and Vegetables

Fruits and vegetables should be the cornerstone of a menopause-friendly diet. They are packed with essential vitamins, minerals, antioxidants, and fiber, all of which play crucial roles in managing menopausal symptoms and promoting overall health. Aim for a vibrant assortment of colors on your plate, as different hues indicate the presence of various beneficial plant compounds. For example, leafy greens like kale and spinach are rich in calcium and folate, while berries and citrus fruits provide a boost of vitamin C and antioxidants.

Diversity in Protein Sources

Protein is essential for maintaining muscle mass, supporting bone health, and promoting satiety. While lean meats, poultry, and fish are excellent protein sources, it's equally important to incorporate plant-based options like legumes, nuts, seeds, and soy products. This variety ensures that you're getting a well-rounded mix of essential amino acids, as well as beneficial nutrients like fiber, healthy fats, and phytoestrogens.

Balance in Carbohydrates

Carbohydrates are a vital source of energy, but it's essential to choose the right types.

opt for complex carbohydrates found in whole grains, starchy vegetables, and legumes, as they provide sustained energy and are rich in fiber, vitamins, and minerals. Limit your intake of refined carbohydrates, such as white bread, pastries, and sugary snacks, as they can contribute to weight gain and blood sugar imbalances.

Healthy Fats for Menopause

Contrary to popular belief, not all fats are created equal. Healthy fats, such as those found in avocados, nuts, seeds, and fatty fish, are essential for hormone regulation, brain function, and heart health. Incorporate a variety of these nutrient-dense fats into your diet, while minimizing your intake of unhealthy saturated and Trans fats found in processed foods and fried items.

Hydration and Fluids

Staying properly hydrated is crucial during menopause, as it can help alleviate symptoms like hot flashes and vaginal dryness. While water should be your primary beverage choice, you can also incorporate other fluids like herbal teas, low-fat milk, and unsweetened juices for added variety and nutrients.

Your menopause-friendly diet will satisfy your nutritional demands and provide you with a varied and pleasant eating experience if you embrace balance and diversity. By using this method, you can be confident that you're giving your body the nutrients it needs to control menopausal symptoms, maintain a healthy weight, and promote general wellbeing. Try new foods, tastes, and dishes without fear; this culinary adventure may be energizing as well as tasty.

Chapter 3: Breakfast Recipes

Chia Seed Pudding

Prep Time: 5 minutes Cooking Time: None (refrigeration for 1-2 hours or overnight) Serving Size: 1 serving

Ingredients:

- 3-4 tablespoons chia seeds
- 1 cup almond milk
- 1-2 tablespoons maple syrup (to taste)
- 1 teaspoon vanilla extract
- Fresh berries for topping

Instructions:

1. In a bowl, combine the chia seeds, almond milk, maple syrup, and vanilla extract.

2. Stir the mixture well to combine.

3. Let it sit for 5 minutes, then stir again to break up any clumps.

4. Cover and refrigerate for 1-2 hours or overnight.

5. Top with fresh berries before serving.

Nutritional Value:

- Calories: 200-300 calories
- Protein: 4-5 grams
- Carbohydrates: 17-24 grams
- Fat: 11-14 grams
- Fiber: 10-15 grams

Quinoa Porridge

Prep Time: 5 minutes Cooking Time: 15-20 minutes
Serving Size: 1 serving

Ingredients:

- ½ cup quinoa
- ¼ teaspoon cinnamon
- 1 ½ cups almond milk
- ½ cup water
- 2 tablespoons maple syrup
- 1 teaspoon vanilla extract
- A pinch of sea salt

Instructions:

1. Rinse quinoa under cold water.

2. In a pot, combine quinoa, cinnamon, almond milk, water, maple syrup, vanilla extract, and sea salt.

3. Bring to a boil, then reduce heat to simmer.

4. Cook for 15-20 minutes, stirring occasionally, until the quinoa is cooked and the mixture has thickened to your liking.

5. Serve warm.

Nutritional Value:

- Calories: 250-350 calories
- Protein: 8-10 grams
- Carbohydrates: 40-50 grams
- Fat: 5-7 grams
- Fiber: 5-7 grams

Avocado Toast

Prep Time: 5 minutes Cooking Time: 1-2 minutes (toasting bread) Serving Size: 1 serving

Ingredients:

- 1 slice whole-grain bread
- ½ ripe avocado
- A sprinkle of feta cheese
- 2-3 cherry tomatoes, halved
- Salt and pepper to taste

Instructions:

1. Toast the bread to your desired level of crispiness.

2. In a bowl, mash the avocado with a fork and season with salt and pepper.

3. Spread the mashed avocado evenly over the toast.

4. Sprinkle feta cheese on top and add the cherry tomato halves.

5. Serve immediately.

Nutritional Value:

- Calories: 200-300 calories
- Protein: 6-8 grams
- Carbohydrates: 20-30 grams
- Fat: 15-20 grams
- Fiber: 7-10 grams

Greek Yogurt Parfait

Prep Time: 10 minutes Cooking Time: No cooking required Serving Size: 1 parfait

Ingredients:

- 1 cup Greek yogurt
- 1/2 cup granola
- 1/4 cup mixed nuts (almonds, walnuts, etc.)
- 1/2 cup seasonal fruits (berries, banana slices, etc.)

Instructions:

1. In a serving glass or bowl, layer 1/3 of the Greek yogurt at the bottom.
2. Add a layer of 1/4 cup of granola.
3. Add a layer of 1/8 cup of mixed nuts.
4. Add a layer of 1/4 cup of seasonal fruits.
5. Repeat the layers until all ingredients are used.

Nutritional Value:

- Calories: 450
- Protein: 25g
- Carbohydrates: 50g
- Fat: 20g
- Fiber: 6g

Spinach and Mushroom Omelette

Prep Time: 5 minutes Cooking Time: 8 minutes
Serving Size: 1 omelette

Ingredients:

- 2 large eggs
- 1 tablespoon milk
- 1/2 cup fresh spinach, chopped
- 1/2 cup mushrooms, sliced
- 1/4 cup cheese, shredded
- Salt and pepper to taste
- 1 teaspoon olive oil

Instructions:

1. In a bowl, whisk together eggs, milk, salt, and pepper.

2. Heat olive oil in a non-stick skillet over medium heat. Sauté mushrooms until browned, then add spinach and cook until wilted.

3. Pour the egg mixture over the vegetables.

4. Sprinkle cheese on one half of the omelette. Once the eggs are set, fold the omelette in half and cook until cheese is melted.

Nutritional Value:

- Calories: 300
- Protein: 20g
- Carbohydrates: 5g
- Fat: 22g Fiber: 1g

Banana Pancakes

Prep Time: 10 minutes Cooking Time: 5 minutes per batch Serving Size: 2 pancakes

Ingredients:

- 1 ripe banana, mashed
- 1 cup whole wheat flour
- 2 large eggs
- 1/2 teaspoon baking powder
- 1/4 cup milk
- 1 tablespoon honey or maple syrup
- Butter or oil for cooking

Instructions:

1. In a mixing bowl, combine mashed banana, eggs, milk, and honey. In another bowl, mix whole wheat flour and baking powder.

2. Combine wet and dry ingredients until just mixed.

3. Heat a lightly oiled griddle or frying pan over medium-high heat.

4. Pour or scoop the batter onto the griddle, using approximately 1/4 cup for each pancake.

5. Cook until pancakes are golden brown on both sides.

Nutritional Value:

- Calories: 350
- Protein: 12g
- Carbohydrates: 60g
- Fat: 8g Fiber: 8g

Savory Muffins

Prep Time: 15 minutes Cooking Time: 20-25 minutes
Serving Size: 1 muffin

Ingredients:

- 2 cups whole wheat flour
- 2 large eggs
- 1 cup milk
- 1/2 cup spinach, chopped
- 1/2 cup onion, diced
- 1/2 cup bell pepper, diced
- 1 teaspoon baking powder
- 1/2 teaspoon salt
- 1/4 teaspoon pepper
- 1/4 cup olive oil

Instructions:

1. Preheat oven to 375°F (190°C) and grease a muffin tin.

2. In a bowl, mix together flour, baking powder, salt, and pepper.

3. In another bowl, whisk eggs, milk, and olive oil.

4. Stir in spinach, onion, and bell pepper.

5. Combine wet and dry ingredients until just mixed.

6. Spoon batter into muffin tins and bake for 20-25 minutes or until a toothpick inserted into the center comes out clean.

Nutritional Value:

- Calories: 180
- Protein: 6g
- Carbohydrates: 24g
- Fat: 7g
- Fiber: 4g

Chapter 4: Lunch Recipes

Mediterranean Quinoa Salad

Prep Time: 15 mins Cooking Time: 15 mins

Ingredients:

- 1 cup quinoa
- 2 cups water
- 1/2 cup diced cucumbers
- 1/2 cup cherry tomatoes, halved
- 1/4 cup diced red onion
- 1/4 cup feta cheese, crumbled
- 1/4 cup kalamata olives, pitted and sliced
- 2 tbsp olive oil
- Juice of 1 lemon
- 1 tsp dried oregano
- Salt and pepper to taste

Instructions:

1. Rinse quinoa under cold water. In a saucepan, bring water to a boil. Add quinoa, reduce heat to low, cover, and simmer for 15 minutes. Fluff quinoa with a fork and allow it to cool. In a large bowl, combine cooled quinoa, cucumbers, tomatoes, red onion, feta cheese, and olives. In a small bowl, whisk together olive oil, lemon juice, oregano, salt, and pepper.

2. Pour dressing over salad and toss to combine. Serve chilled or at room temperature.

Curried Lentil Soup

Prep Time: 10 mins Cooking Time: 30 mins

Ingredients:

- 1 tbsp olive oil
- 1 onion, chopped
- 2 cloves garlic, minced
- 1 tbsp curry powder
- 1 cup red lentils
- 4 cups vegetable broth
- 1 can (14 oz) diced tomatoes
- Salt and pepper to taste

Instructions:

1. Heat oil in a large pot over medium heat. Add onion and garlic, cook until softened.
2. Stir in curry powder and cook for another minute.
3. Add lentils, broth, and tomatoes. Bring to a boil, then reduce heat and simmer for 30 minutes.
4. Season with salt and pepper. Serve hot.

Grilled Veggie Wrap

Prep Time: 20 mins Cooking Time: 10 mins

Ingredients:

- 1 zucchini, sliced
- 1 bell pepper, sliced
- 1 red onion, sliced
- 2 tbsp balsamic vinegar
- 1 tbsp olive oil
- Salt and pepper to taste
- 4 whole wheat wraps
- 1/2 cup hummus
- 1/2 cup goat cheese, crumbled

Instructions:

1. Preheat grill to medium-high heat.

2. Toss zucchini, bell pepper, and red onion with balsamic vinegar, olive oil, salt, and pepper.

3. Grill vegetables until tender and slightly charred.

4. Spread hummus on wraps, add grilled vegetables and goat cheese.

5. Roll up wraps tightly, cut in half, and serve.

Tofu Stir-Fry

Prep Time: 15 mins Cooking Time: 10 mins

Ingredients:

- 1 block firm tofu, drained and cubed
- 2 tbsp soy sauce
- 1 tbsp sesame oil
- 1 tbsp cornstarch
- 2 cups mixed vegetables (broccoli, bell peppers, carrots)
- 2 cloves garlic, minced
- 1 tbsp ginger, minced
- 2 tbsp vegetable oil

Instructions:

1. Toss tofu with soy sauce, sesame oil, and cornstarch.

2. Heat vegetable oil in a pan over medium-high heat. Add tofu and cook until golden brown.

3. Add garlic, ginger, and vegetables. Stir-fry until vegetables are tender.

4. Serve hot with rice or noodles.

Chickpea Salad Sandwich

Prep Time: 15 mins Cooking Time: 0 mins

Ingredients:

- 1 can (15 oz) chickpeas, drained and rinsed
- 1/4 cup vegan mayonnaise
- 1 tbsp Dijon mustard
- 1/2 tsp garlic powder
- 1/2 tsp onion powder
- Salt and pepper to taste
- 1 tbsp fresh dill, chopped
- Bread slices
- Lettuce leaves

Instructions:

1. Mash chickpeas in a bowl using a fork or potato masher.

2. Stir in vegan mayonnaise, Dijon mustard, garlic powder, onion powder, salt, pepper, and dill.

3. Spread chickpea mixture onto bread slices, top with lettuce, and assemble the sandwich.

Stuffed Bell Peppers

Prep Time: 20 mins Cooking Time: 1 hr

Ingredients:

- 6 large bell peppers (any color)
- 1 pound ground beef
- 1 onion, chopped
- 2 cloves garlic, minced
- 1 cup cooked rice
- 1 cup tomato sauce
- 1/2 cup shredded cheese (e.g., cheddar or mozzarella)
- 1 tsp salt
- 1/2 tsp pepper
- 1 tsp Italian seasoning

Instructions:

1. Preheat oven to 350°F (175°C).

2. Cut the tops off the peppers and remove the seeds.

3. In a skillet, cook ground beef, onion, and garlic over medium heat until beef is browned; drain.

4. Stir in rice, 1/2 cup tomato sauce, salt, pepper, and Italian seasoning. Stuff each bell pepper with the beef mixture and place in a baking dish.

5. Pour the remaining tomato sauce over the stuffed peppers. Bake in the preheated oven for 45 minutes.

6. Sprinkle shredded cheese on top of each pepper and bake for an additional 15 minutes, or until the cheese is melted and bubbly.

Black Bean Taco Salad

Prep Time: 15 mins Cooking Time: 0 mins

Ingredients:

- 4 cups romaine lettuce, chopped
- 1 can (15 oz) black beans, rinsed and drained
- 1 can (15 oz) corn, drained
- 1 cup cherry tomatoes, halved
- 1/2 cup cheddar cheese, shredded
- 1/3 cup green onions, chopped
- 1/3 cup tortilla chips, crushed

For the dressing:

- 1/2 cup sour cream
- 1/4 cup salsa
- 1/2 tsp ground cumin
- Juice of 1/2 a lime
- Salt, to taste

Instructions:

1. In a small bowl, whisk together the sour cream, salsa, cumin, lime juice, and salt to create the dressing.

2. In a large bowl, combine the lettuce, black beans, corn, tomatoes, green onions, and half of the cheddar cheese. Pour the dressing over the salad and toss to

coat evenly. Top with the remaining cheddar cheese
and crushed tortilla chips. Serve immediately or chill
in the refrigerator until ready to serve.

Chapter 5: Dinner Recipes

Eggplant Chickpea Curry

Prep Time: 20 mins Cooking Time: 40 mins

Ingredients:

- 1 large eggplant, diced
- 1 can chickpeas, drained
- 1 onion, chopped
- 2 cloves garlic, minced
- 1 tbsp curry powder
- 1 tsp cumin
- 1 tsp turmeric
- 1/2 tsp cayenne pepper
- Salt to taste
- 2 cups diced tomatoes
- 1 cup coconut milk
- Fresh cilantro for garnish

Instructions:

1. Preheat the oven to 400°F (200°C). Place diced eggplant on a baking sheet, drizzle with oil, and roast for 20 minutes.

2. Sauté onion and garlic in a large pan until translucent. Add spices and cook for another minute.

3. Stir in roasted eggplant, chickpeas, tomatoes, and coconut milk. Simmer for 20 minutes.

4. Garnish with cilantro and serve with rice or naan.

Baked Salmon with Dill

Prep Time: 10 mins Cooking Time: 25 mins

Ingredients:

- 4 salmon fillets
- 2 tbsp olive oil
- 2 tbsp fresh dill, chopped
- 1 lemon, juice and zest
- Salt and pepper to taste

Instructions:

1. Preheat oven to 350°F (175°C).

2. Place salmon on a baking sheet lined with parchment paper.

3. Mix olive oil, dill, lemon juice, zest, salt, and pepper. Brush over salmon.

4. Bake for 20-25 minutes or until salmon flakes easily.

Roasted Cauliflower Steaks

Prep Time: 10 mins Cooking Time: 30 mins

Ingredients:

- 1 large head cauliflower
- 2 tbsp olive oil
- 1 tbsp lemon juice
- 2 cloves garlic, minced
- Red pepper flakes to taste
- Salt and pepper to taste

Instructions:

1. Preheat oven to 400°F (200°C).

2. Slice cauliflower into 1-inch-thick steaks. Place on a baking sheet.

3. Whisk together olive oil, lemon juice, garlic, red pepper flakes, salt, and pepper. Brush mixture over cauliflower.

4. Roast for 30 minutes or until tender and golden.

Lemon Herb Chicken Breast

Prep Time: 15 mins Cooking Time: 10 mins

Ingredients:

- 4 chicken breasts
- 2 tbsp olive oil
- 1 lemon, juice and zest
- 1 tbsp mixed dried herbs (oregano, thyme, parsley)
- 2 cloves garlic, minced
- Salt and pepper to taste

Instructions:

1. Marinate chicken with olive oil, lemon juice, zest, herbs, garlic, salt, and pepper for at least 30 minutes.

2. Preheat a grill or skillet over medium-high heat.

3. Cook chicken for 5 minutes on each side or until internal temperature reaches 165°F (75°C).

Garlic Green Beans

Prep Time: 5 mins Cooking Time: 10 mins

Ingredients:

- 1 lb green beans, trimmed
- 2 tbsp butter
- 3 cloves garlic, minced
- Salt and pepper to taste

Instructions:

1. Blanch green beans in boiling water for 3 minutes, then transfer to ice water.

2. Melt butter in a pan over medium heat. Add garlic and cook until fragrant.

3. Add green beans, salt, and pepper. Sauté until coated and heated through.

Spaghetti Squash Primavera

Prep Time: 15 mins Cooking Time: 45 mins

Ingredients:

- 1 spaghetti squash
- 2 tbsp olive oil
- 1 onion, chopped
- 1 zucchini, diced
- 1 bell pepper, chopped
- 1 cup cherry tomatoes, halved
- 1/2 cup feta cheese, crumbled
- 1 tbsp Italian seasoning
- Salt and pepper to taste

Instructions:

1. Microwave spaghetti squash for 12 minutes, then cut in half, remove seeds, and shred with a fork.

2. Sauté onion, zucchini, and bell pepper with Italian seasoning and salt and pepper.

3. Add tomatoes and cook until warmed. Mix in spaghetti squash strands and feta cheese.

Quinoa Stuffed Tomatoes

Prep Time: 20 mins Cooking Time: 20 mins

Ingredients:

- 8 large tomatoes
- 1 cup cooked quinoa
- 1/2 cup feta cheese, crumbled
- 1/4 cup fresh basil, chopped
- 2 tbsp pine nuts
- Salt and pepper to taste

Instructions:

1. Preheat oven to 375°F (190°C).

2. Cut tops off tomatoes and scoop out insides.

3. Mix quinoa, feta, basil, pine nuts, salt, and pepper. Stuff mixture into tomatoes.

4. Bake for 20 minutes or until tomatoes are tender.

Chapter 6: Snacks and Desserts

Almond Butter Energy Balls

Prep Time: 10 mins

Ingredients:

- 1 cup almond butter
- 1/4 cup honey or maple syrup
- 1/2 cup rolled oats
- 1/2 cup mini chocolate chips
- 1/4 cup ground flaxseed
- Pinch of salt

Instructions:

1. In a bowl, mix together almond butter and honey until well combined.

2. Add in oats, chocolate chips, flaxseed, and salt. Stir until the mixture is well mixed.

3. Roll the mixture into 1-inch balls and place on a baking sheet lined with parchment paper.

4. Refrigerate for at least 30 minutes before serving.

Carrot Cake Oatmeal Cookies

Prep Time: 15 mins Cooking Time: 20 mins

Ingredients:

- 3/4 cup melted butter
- 3/4 cup brown sugar
- 1 large egg
- 1 cup shredded carrots
- 2 cups rolled oats
- 1 teaspoon baking soda
- 1/2 teaspoon ground cinnamon

Instructions:

1. Preheat oven to 375°F (190°C). Grease baking sheets.

2. Beat together butter, brown sugar, egg, and add carrots.

3. Mix in oats, baking soda, and cinnamon.

4. Drop by teaspoonfuls onto prepared baking sheets and bake until golden.

Dark Chocolate Avocado Truffles

Prep Time: 10 mins Chill Time: 20 mins

Ingredients:

- 1 ripe avocado
- 1/2 cup dark chocolate chips
- Cocoa powder for coating

Instructions:

1. Mash avocado until smooth.

2. Melt chocolate chips and mix with avocado until combined.

3. Chill mixture for 20 minutes, then form into balls and roll in cocoa powder.

Baked Apple Chips

Prep Time: 10 mins Cooking Time: 2 hrs

Ingredients:

- 2 tablespoons sugar
- 1 tablespoon ground cinnamon
- 4 apples, thinly sliced

Instructions:

1. Preheat oven to 250°F (120°C). Line baking sheets with parchment paper.

2. Mix sugar and cinnamon, toss with apple slices.

3. Bake until edges are crisp, about 2 hours.

Pumpkin Seed Granola Bars

Prep Time: 10 mins Cooking Time: 22 mins

Ingredients:

- 1/4 cup honey
- 1/2 teaspoon vanilla extract
- 1/4 cup almond meal
- 1 teaspoon pumpkin pie spice
- 1 Tablespoon almond butter
- 1 and 1/3 cups almonds, chopped
- 1/2 cup dried cranberries
- 3/4 cup pumpkin seeds

Instructions:

1. Mix honey, vanilla, almond meal, spice, and almond butter.
2. Add almonds, cranberries, and pumpkin seeds.
3. Press into a pan and bake for 22 minutes.

Coconut Yogurt Popsicles

Prep Time: 5 mins

Ingredients:

- Coconut milk
- Yogurt
- Sweetener of choice
- Optional: fruits or flavors

Instructions:

1. Blend coconut milk, yogurt, and sweetener.
2. Pour into Popsicle molds and freeze until solid.

Raspberry Chia Pudding

Prep Time: 10 mins Chill Time: 3 hrs

Ingredients:

- Milk of choice
- Raspberries
- Maple syrup
- Vanilla extract
- Chia seeds

Instructions:

1. Blend milk, raspberries, syrup, and vanilla.
2. Stir in chia seeds and refrigerate until set.

Walnut-Stuffed Dates

Prep Time: 10 mins

Ingredients:

- Medjool dates
- Walnut halves
- Optional: chocolate chips, honey, cocoa, cinnamon

Instructions:

1. Slice dates and remove pits.
2. Stuff with walnuts and optional ingredients.
3. Serve as is or chilled.

Chapter 7: Meal Plan Chapter

Sample weekly meal plans

Week 1 Meal Plan

Monday:

- Breakfast: Smoothie Bowl
- Lunch: Mediterranean Quinoa Salad
- Dinner: Eggplant Chickpea Curry
- Snack: Almond Butter Energy Balls

Tuesday:

- Breakfast: Overnight Oats
- Lunch: Curried Lentil Soup
- Dinner: Baked Salmon with Dill
- Snack: Carrot Cake Oatmeal Cookies

Wednesday:

- Breakfast: Chia Seed Pudding
- Lunch: Grilled Veggie Wrap
- Dinner: Roasted Cauliflower Steaks
- Snack: Dark Chocolate Avocado Truffles

Thursday:

- Breakfast: Quinoa Porridge
- Lunch: Chickpea Salad Sandwich
- Dinner: Lemon Herb Chicken Breast
- Snack: Baked Apple Chips

Friday:

- Breakfast: Avocado Toast
- Lunch: Stuffed Bell Peppers
- Dinner: Garlic Green Beans
- Snack: Pumpkin Seed Granola Bars

Saturday:

- Breakfast: Greek Yogurt Parfait
- Lunch: Black Bean Taco Salad
- Dinner: Spaghetti Squash Primavera
- Snack: Coconut Yogurt Popsicles

Sunday:

- Breakfast: Spinach and Mushroom Omelette
- Lunch: Tofu Stir-Fry
- Dinner: Quinoa Stuffed Tomatoes
- Snack: Raspberry Chia Pudding

Week 2 Meal Plan

Monday:

- Breakfast: Banana Pancakes
- Lunch: Mediterranean Quinoa Salad
- Dinner: Eggplant Chickpea Curry
- Snack: Walnut-Stuffed Dates

Tuesday:

- Breakfast: Smoothie Bowl
- Lunch: Curried Lentil Soup
- Dinner: Baked Salmon with Dill
- Snack: Almond Butter Energy Balls

Wednesday:

- Breakfast: Overnight Oats
- Lunch: Grilled Veggie Wrap
- Dinner: Roasted Cauliflower Steaks
- Snack: Carrot Cake Oatmeal Cookies

Thursday:

- Breakfast: Chia Seed Pudding
- Lunch: Chickpea Salad Sandwich
- Dinner: Lemon Herb Chicken Breast
- Snack: Dark Chocolate Avocado Truffles

Friday:

- Breakfast: Quinoa Porridge
- Lunch: Stuffed Bell Peppers
- Dinner: Garlic Green Beans
- Snack: Baked Apple Chips

Saturday:

- Breakfast: Avocado Toast
- Lunch: Black Bean Taco Salad
- Dinner: Spaghetti Squash Primavera
- Snack: Pumpkin Seed Granola Bars

Sunday:

- Breakfast: Greek Yogurt Parfait
- Lunch: Tofu Stir-Fry
- Dinner: Quinoa Stuffed Tomatoes
- Snack: Coconut Yogurt Popsicles

Week 3 Meal Plan

Monday:
- Breakfast: Spinach and Mushroom Omelette
- Lunch: Mediterranean Quinoa Salad
- Dinner: Eggplant Chickpea Curry
- Snack: Raspberry Chia Pudding

Tuesday:
- Breakfast: Banana Pancakes
- Lunch: Curried Lentil Soup
- Dinner: Baked Salmon with Dill
- Snack: Walnut-Stuffed Dates

Wednesday:
- Breakfast: Smoothie Bowl
- Lunch: Grilled Veggie Wrap
- Dinner: Roasted Cauliflower Steaks
- Snack: Almond Butter Energy Balls

Thursday:
- Breakfast: Overnight Oats
- Lunch: Chickpea Salad Sandwich
- Dinner: Lemon Herb Chicken Breast
- Snack: Carrot Cake Oatmeal Cookies

Friday:
- Breakfast: Chia Seed Pudding
- Lunch: Stuffed Bell Peppers
- Dinner: Garlic Green Beans
- Snack: Dark Chocolate Avocado Truffles

Saturday:

- Breakfast: Quinoa Porridge
- Lunch: Black Bean Taco Salad
- Dinner: Spaghetti Squash Primavera
- Snack: Baked Apple Chips

Sunday:

- Breakfast: Avocado Toast
- Lunch: Tofu Stir-Fry
- Dinner: Quinoa Stuffed Tomatoes
- Snack: Pumpkin Seed Granola Bars

Tips for Meal Preparation and Planning

Meal preparation and planning are the cornerstones of a successful diet, especially during menopause. This phase of life brings about various changes in the body, and a well-thought-out meal plan can help manage symptoms and maintain health. The following tips will help you navigate this process with ease and confidence.

Understanding Your Nutritional Needs

Menopause alters your body's nutritional requirements. It's crucial to understand these changes to prepare meals that support your health. Focus on calcium for bone health, omega-3 fatty acids for heart health, and fiber for digestive wellness. Incorporate foods rich in these nutrients into your weekly meal plans.

Planning Your Meals

1. Start with a Calendar: Use a calendar to plan your meals for the week. This visual aid will help you organize your thoughts and ensure variety in your diet.

2. Balance Your Plate: Aim for a balance of lean proteins, whole grains, healthy fats, and plenty of fruits and vegetables.

3. Consider Portion Sizes: Menopause can slow down metabolism, so be mindful of portion sizes to avoid unwanted weight gain.

4. Plan for Snacks: Healthy snacking can keep your energy levels up and prevent overeating at meal times.

Preparation Tips

1. Cook in Batches: Prepare larger portions of versatile ingredients like quinoa or roasted vegetables to use in different meals throughout the week.

2. Use Healthy Cooking Methods: Opt for baking, steaming, or grilling rather than frying to reduce fat intake.

3. Season Smartly: Use herbs and spices to add flavor without extra salt or sugar.

4. Embrace Leftovers: Plan to have leftovers from dinner for lunch the next day to save time and effort.

Time-Saving Strategies

1. Prep Ingredients Ahead: Wash and chop vegetables, marinate proteins, and measure out dry ingredients in advance.

2. Invest in Quality Containers: Store prepped ingredients and leftovers in clear, airtight containers for easy access and freshness.

3. Schedule Prep Time: Set aside a few hours each week to focus on meal prep. This can be a relaxing and productive part of your routine.

Staying Flexible

Life is unpredictable, and so is appetite. Have backup plans for days when cooking isn't feasible, like healthy frozen meals or quick recipes that require minimal effort.

Grocery Shopping Made Easy

1. Make a List: Always shop with a list to avoid impulse buys and ensure you have all the ingredients you need.
2. Shop the Perimeter: The outer aisles of the grocery store typically contain the freshest, most nutritious foods.
3. Read Labels: Pay attention to food labels to choose items with less added sugar, salt, and unhealthy fats.

Grocery Lists and Pantry Essentials

A well-stocked pantry and a smart grocery list are your best allies in maintaining a healthy menopause diet. They ensure that you have all the necessary ingredients on hand to prepare nutritious meals and snacks.

Building Your Grocery List

Your grocery list should reflect the meals you've planned for the week. Group items by category to make shopping more efficient. Include a variety of:

- Fresh fruits and vegetables
- Lean proteins like fish, poultry, and legumes
- Whole grains such as brown rice, quinoa, and whole wheat pasta
- Low-fat dairy or dairy alternatives
- Healthy fats like avocados, nuts, and olive oil

Pantry Essentials

Stock your pantry with items that have a longer shelf life and can be used in multiple recipes:

- Canned goods: beans, tomatoes, and fish
- Whole grains: oats, quinoa, and barley
- Nuts and seeds: almonds, chia seeds, and flaxseeds
- Spices and herbs: basil, cumin, and turmeric
- Oils and vinegars: extra virgin olive oil and balsamic vinegar
- Condiments: mustard, low-sodium soy sauce, and salsa

Refrigerator and Freezer Staples

Keep your refrigerator and freezer filled with:

- Fresh produce: leafy greens, berries, and cruciferous vegetables
- Proteins: eggs, Greek yogurt, and tofu
- Frozen items: mixed vegetables, berries, and shrimp

By following these tips for meal preparation and planning, along with keeping a well-stocked kitchen, you'll be well on your way to a healthier menopause experience. Remember, the key is to plan ahead, stay organized, and be flexible. With these strategies in place, you'll find that eating well can be both simple and satisfying.

Chapter 8: Understanding Menopause Symptoms

Menopause is a complicated journey that impacts many facets of a woman's life rather than just being a biological occurrence. The decrease in estrogen and progesterone levels that occurs as the body moves away from its reproductive phase may cause a variety of symptoms that vary in degree and duration. This chapter examines these symptoms in detail and shows how nutrition may be a key factor in controlling them.

The Menopause Transition

Understanding the stages of menopause is crucial. The transition typically begins with perimenopause, where cycles become irregular. This phase can last for several years before reaching menopause, which is followed by postmenopause, marking the end of menstrual periods.

Common Menopause Symptoms

Hot Flashes and Night Sweats

One of the most noticeable and troublesome menopausal symptoms is the onset of hot flashes. They can strike at any time, causing intense heat, flushing, and perspiration. Night sweats may disrupt sleep, leading to fatigue and irritability.

Mood Changes

Hormonal fluctuations can significantly impact mood. Women may experience heightened emotions, anxiety, and depression. These mood changes are not only distressing but can also strain personal relationships and affect daily functioning.

Sleep Problems

Quality sleep becomes elusive for many during menopause. Insomnia, frequent awakenings, and difficulty falling asleep are common complaints. Poor sleep can exacerbate other menopause symptoms and affect overall health.

Weight Gain and Slowed Metabolism

Many women notice a shift in their body composition during menopause, with increased fat accumulation around the midsection. A slower metabolism can make weight management more challenging.

Thinning Hair and Dry Skin

Estrogen plays a role in maintaining skin elasticity and hair strength. As levels decline, women may notice their skin becoming drier and less supple, and their hair may thin or become brittle.

Vaginal Dryness

Reduced estrogen can lead to vaginal atrophy, characterized by dryness, itching, and discomfort. This condition can affect intimate relationships and lead to a decrease in sexual well-being.

Loss of Breast Fullness

Changes in breast tissue can result in a loss of fullness and firmness. This physical change is a direct result of hormonal shifts and can affect body image and self-esteem.

Dietary Approaches to Manage Specific Symptoms

For Hot Flashes and Night Sweats

Dietary adjustments can help manage these temperature fluctuations. Phytoestrogens found in soy products mimic estrogen and may offer relief. Flaxseed, with its lignans, can also have a beneficial effect. Vitamin E-rich foods like almonds and spinach might provide some women with respite from hot flashes.

For Mood Changes

Omega-3 fatty acids are known for their mood-stabilizing effects. Incorporating fish, flaxseeds, and walnuts into the diet can support emotional well-being. Complex carbohydrates from whole grains promote steady blood sugar levels, which can help stabilize mood. B vitamins, particularly B6 and B12, are vital for the production of neurotransmitters like serotonin and dopamine, which regulate mood.

For Sleep Problems

Magnesium plays a role in muscle relaxation and nerve function, which can aid sleep. Foods rich in magnesium, such as leafy greens and legumes, should be a staple in the diet.

Herbal teas like chamomile and valerian root can also promote relaxation and improve sleep quality.

For Weight Gain and Slowed Metabolism

A diet high in fiber can enhance feelings of fullness and aid digestion, helping to manage weight. Lean proteins, including chicken, fish, and plant-based options like lentils, can increase metabolism and support muscle mass.

For Thinning Hair and Dry Skin

The formation of collagen, which is beneficial to skin health, requires vitamin C. Zinc helps hair growth and repair. Including a mix of fruits, vegetables, and lean meats can give these nutrients.

For Vaginal Dryness

Staying hydrated is key. Water-rich foods can help maintain hydration. Vitamin A and beta-carotene support the health of mucous membranes and can be found in colorful fruits and vegetables.

For Loss of Breast Fullness

Healthy fats, such as those found in avocados and olive oil, are important for maintaining healthy skin and tissues. Ensuring an adequate intake of these fats can support overall skin health.

Although menopause is a normal aspect of aging, quality of life need not be negatively impacted. Through knowledge of the signs and how to control them with food, women may empower themselves to go through this change with grace and energy. The dietary approaches discussed in this chapter support long-term health and wellbeing in addition to helping with symptom management.

Chapter 9: Lifestyle Strategies for Menopause

While a menopause-friendly diet plays a pivotal role in managing symptoms and promoting overall well-being, it's essential to recognize that a holistic approach is key to thriving during this transitional phase. Embracing a comprehensive lifestyle strategy that encompasses exercise, stress management techniques, and complementary therapies can significantly enhance your journey through menopause. In this chapter, we'll explore these vital elements and provide practical recommendations to help you feel your best.

Exercise Recommendations

Regular physical activity is an invaluable component of a well-rounded menopause management plan. Exercise not only supports weight management and bone health but also contributes to better sleep, reduced stress levels, and an improved overall sense of well-being. Here are some exercise recommendations to consider:

1. Weight-bearing and Resistance Training

As women age and estrogen levels decline, bone loss can become a significant concern, increasing the risk of osteoporosis. Weight-bearing exercises, such as walking, jogging, dancing, and weightlifting, put stress on the bones, prompting them to rebuild and strengthen. Aim for at least two to three sessions of weight-bearing and resistance training per week to maintain bone density and muscle mass.

2. Cardiovascular Exercise

Menopause can increase the risk of heart disease, making regular cardiovascular exercise crucial. Engage in activities that get your heart rate up, such as brisk walking, swimming, cycling, or aerobic classes. Aim for at least 150 minutes of moderate-intensity cardio or 75 minutes of vigorous-intensity cardio per week, spread out over multiple sessions.

3. Mind-Body Exercises

Practices like yoga, tai chi, and Pilates can be excellent additions to your exercise routine. Not only do they promote flexibility, balance, and strength, but they also encourage mindfulness and relaxation, which can help alleviate stress and anxiety – common challenges during menopause.

Menopause can contribute to weakening of the pelvic floor muscles, potentially leading to issues like urinary incontinence. Incorporate pelvic floor exercises, also known as Kegel exercises, into your routine to help strengthen these muscles and improve bladder control.

Recall that if you're new to exercising, it's essential to pay attention to your body and start out carefully. To create an exercise program that is safe and appropriate for you, speak with a medical practitioner or a qualified fitness trainer.

Stress Management Techniques

The hormonal changes during menopause can elevate stress levels, which can, in turn, worsen menopausal symptoms including hot flashes, mood swings, and sleep difficulties. Incorporating stress management practices into your daily routine will help you handle this change with greater ease and resilience. Here are some strategies to consider:

1.   Mindfulness   and   Meditation
Practices like mindfulness meditation, deep breathing exercises, and guided imagery can help quiet the mind, reduce anxiety, and foster a sense of inner peace.

Even just a few minutes of mindfulness meditation each day can have considerable advantages for stress reduction.

2. Yoga and Tai Chi

In addition to their physical benefits, practices like yoga and tai chi can be powerful stress-relieving tools. The combination of gentle movements, controlled breathing, and mindfulness can help quiet the mind and cultivate a sense of tranquility.

3. Journaling and Expressive Writing

Keeping a journal or engaging in expressive writing can be a therapeutic way to process thoughts and emotions during this transitional phase. Writing can provide a safe outlet for stress and help you gain clarity and perspective.

4. Social Support

Building a strong social support system can be invaluable during menopause. Surrounding yourself with understanding friends, family members, or support groups can provide a sense of community, validation, and encouragement as you navigate this journey.

Feeling overwhelmed or overburdened can contribute significantly to stress levels. Practice effective time management strategies, learn to delegate tasks when possible, and prioritize self-care activities to maintain a healthy work-life balance.

Complementary Therapies

In addition to a balanced diet, regular exercise, and stress management techniques, complementary therapies can be valuable adjuncts to your menopause management plan. These alternative approaches may help alleviate specific symptoms and promote overall well-being. However, it's essential to consult with a qualified healthcare professional before incorporating any new therapies, as some may interact with medications or have potential side effects.

1. Herbal Remedies

Certain herbs and botanical supplements have been traditionally used to help manage menopausal symptoms. Black cohosh, for example, has been studied for its potential in reducing hot flashes and night sweats, while red clover and evening primrose oil may help alleviate vaginal dryness.

It's crucial to discuss the safety and efficacy of any herbal remedies with your healthcare provider.

2. Acupuncture

This ancient Chinese practice involves the insertion of thin needles into specific points on the body to promote energy flow and balance. Some women find acupuncture helpful in reducing hot flashes, improving sleep quality, and alleviating other menopausal symptoms.

3. Massage Therapy

Regular massage therapy can promote relaxation, reduce muscle tension, and improve circulation. It may also help alleviate certain menopausal symptoms like joint pain, headaches, and stress-related issues.

4. Aromatherapy

The use of essential oils, such as lavender, clary sage, and geranium, can create a calming and soothing environment. Some women find that aromatherapy helps reduce stress, improve sleep, and alleviate mood-related symptoms associated with menopause.

5. Cognitive-Behavioral Therapy (CBT)

CBT is a form of psychotherapy that can help identify and change negative thought patterns and behaviors.

It may be particularly beneficial for managing menopausal symptoms like anxiety, depression, and stress-related issues.

It's important to remember that every woman's experience with menopause is unique, and what works for one individual may not be effective for another. Be open to exploring different lifestyle strategies and complementary therapies, and don't hesitate to seek guidance from qualified healthcare professionals to find the right combination of approaches that best supports your overall well-being during this transformative phase.

Conclusion

As you reach the end of this comprehensive guide, we hope you feel empowered with the knowledge and tools necessary to navigate menopause with confidence and vitality. By embracing a menopause-friendly dietary approach and integrating lifestyle strategies that promote overall well-being, you've taken a significant step towards reclaiming control over this natural transition.

Throughout these pages, we've explored the intricate connection between nutrition and menopause, delving into the specific ways in which a well-balanced, nutrient-dense diet can alleviate and manage common symptoms like hot flashes, mood changes, weight fluctuations, and bone health concerns. From phytoestrogen-rich foods that mimic the effects of estrogen to calcium-rich sources that support strong bones, and anti-inflammatory ingredients that soothe discomfort, the recipes and meal plans provided have been thoughtfully crafted to nourish your body during this transformative phase.

But our journey didn't stop at diet alone. We recognized the importance of adopting a holistic approach, addressing exercise, stress management, and complementary therapies as vital components of a comprehensive menopause management strategy. By incorporating regular physical activity, mindfulness practices, and exploring alternative modalities like acupuncture or aromatherapy, you've equipped yourself with a well-rounded toolkit to support your physical, mental, and emotional well-being.

As you embark on this new chapter, remember that menopause is a natural process, not a disorder or a disease. Embrace it with a sense of empowerment and self-compassion, recognizing that every woman's experience is unique and valid. The strategies outlined in this book are merely a starting point, a foundation upon which you can build and customize your journey to suit your individual needs and preferences.

We encourage you to continue exploring, experimenting, and fine-tuning your approach until you find the perfect balance that resonates with your mind, body, and spirit. Share your experiences with others, seek guidance from trusted healthcare professionals, and celebrate the small victories along the way – for they are stepping stones towards a more vibrant, fulfilling life during and beyond menopause.

Remember, this transition is not a destination, but rather an opportunity for growth, self-discovery, and newfound resilience. Embrace the wisdom that comes with this phase, and let it inspire you to live your best life, free from the constraints of menopausal symptoms.

We hope that "The New Menopause Diet Cookbook" has served as a valuable companion on this journey, providing practical guidance, delicious recipes, and a sense of empowerment that will carry you through menopause and into the next chapter of your life with grace and confidence.

As we bid farewell, we kindly ask our readers to share their thoughts and experiences with us. Your feedback, insights, and personal stories are invaluable in helping us continue to refine and improve our approach to menopause management. Together, we can create a supportive community that celebrates this transformative phase and empowers women to thrive in every aspect of their lives.

Thank you for joining us on this journey. May the knowledge and tools you've acquired serve as a foundation for a lifetime of vibrant, nourishing experiences that honor the remarkable strength and resilience of the female body and spirit.